Self Care Activities

Edition 2

BOOKLET

WOMAN

Overcoming Self-Doubt and Negativity
I refuse to let myself be the only one who holds
me back. It's time to break free from my own
self-imposed limitations and start thriving.

Sharon McLaurin

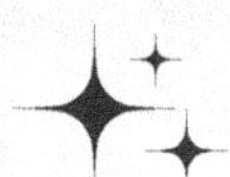

Table of Contents

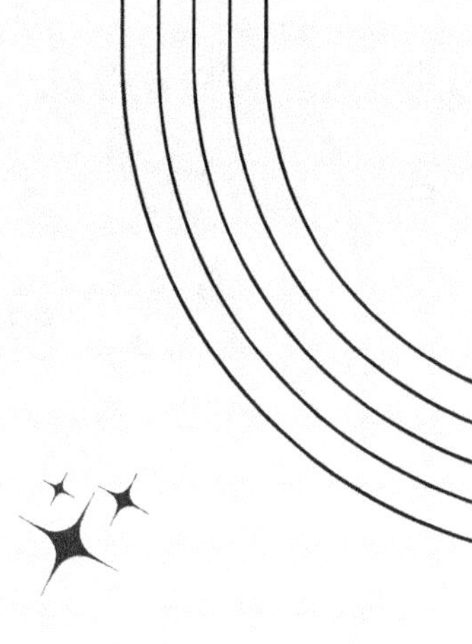

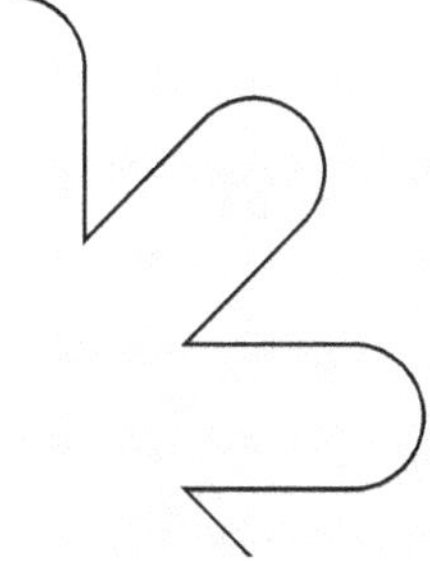

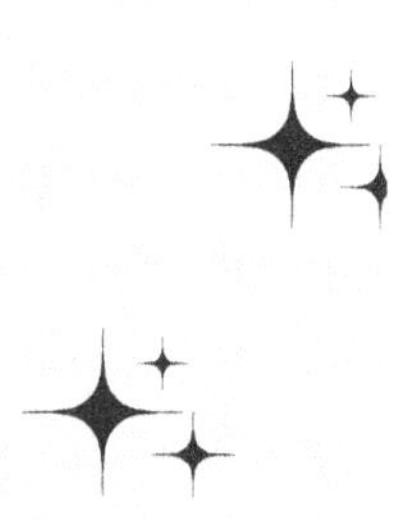

Introduction

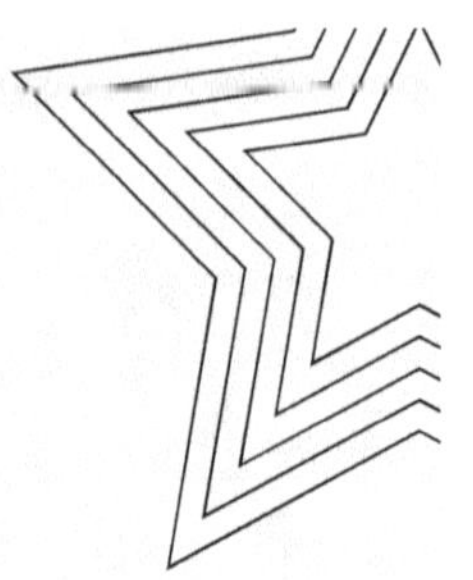

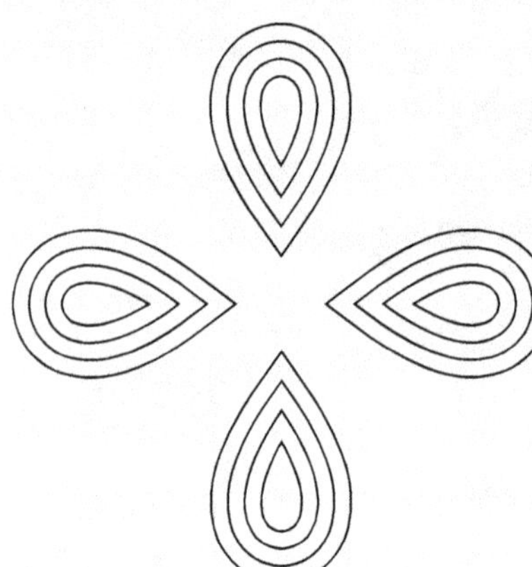

OUR REASONS

Taking care of yourself is a must-do, but when the to-do list is as long as a giraffe's neck, it's easy to forget. Every task needs to have a purpose, right down to the nitty-gritty details. So, unless it's beneficial, why bother doing it?

Disclaimer

The content in this booklet is not intended to be a substitute for professional medical advice, diagnosis, or treatment. Always consult with a qualified and licensed physician or other medical care provider, and follow their advice without delay regardless of anything read in this booklet.

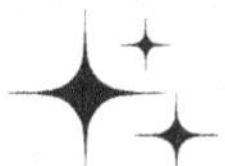

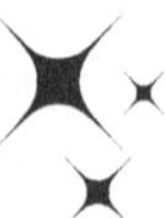

Creating a Self Care Plan

Goals For My Mind

- Wander in the city
- Unplug for an hour
- Keep an journal
- Have a self date
- Go cloud watching
- Do a mini declutter

Goals For My Body

- Take a few deep breaths
- Run for a few minutes
- Take a quick nap
- Have a good laugh
- Do a massage
- Wake up at 6

MIND

BODY

NOTES

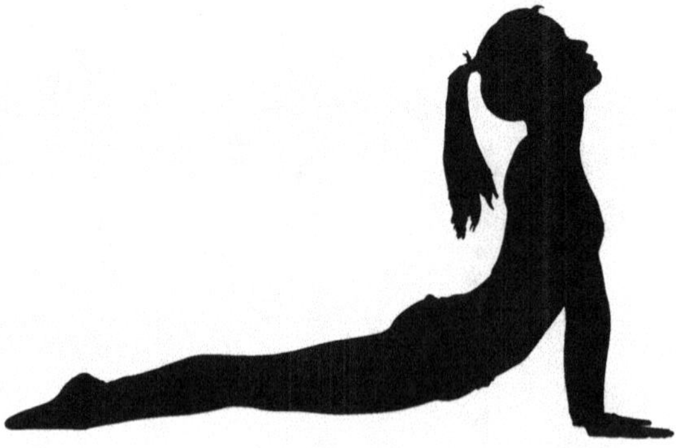

NOTES

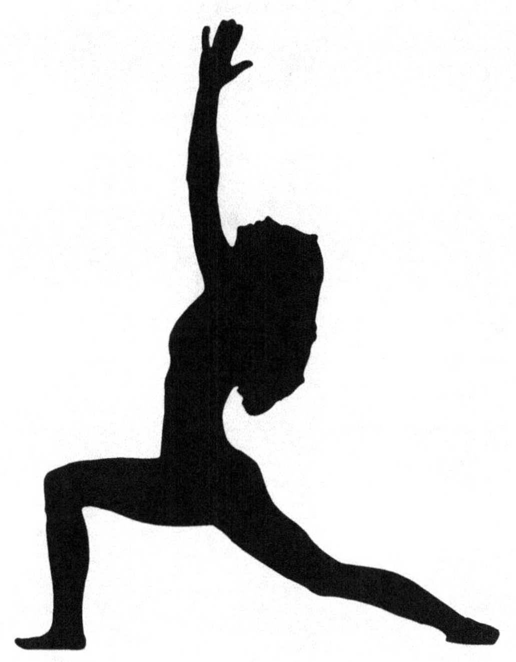

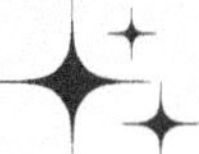

Understanding Self Care

WHAT IS SELF CARE?

Self care is an activity carried out by individuals to care for themselves with things that benefit themselves, both spiritually and physically. In short, self care is taking care of yourself.

However, self care is often considered selfish by some people. Why is that? This happens because from a young age our mindset or some people have been taught that "we have to care about and prioritize other people before ourselves." Finally, the concept is embedded by some people.

Indeed, caring and being concerned about others is something that needs to be applied within yourself, but don't forget to remain selfish. In fact, self care must be balanced.

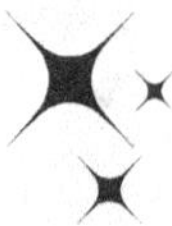

NOTES

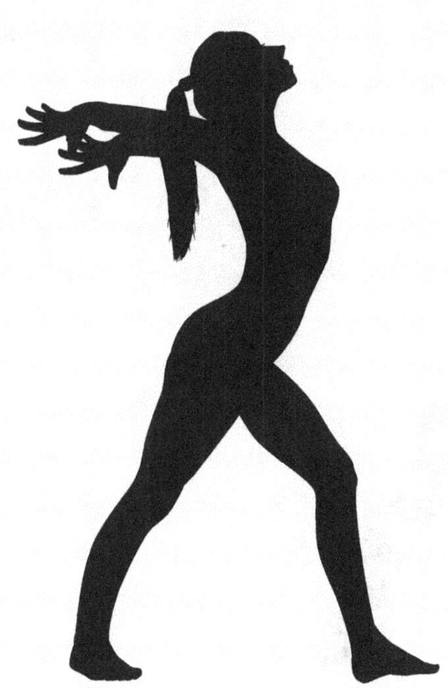

NOTES

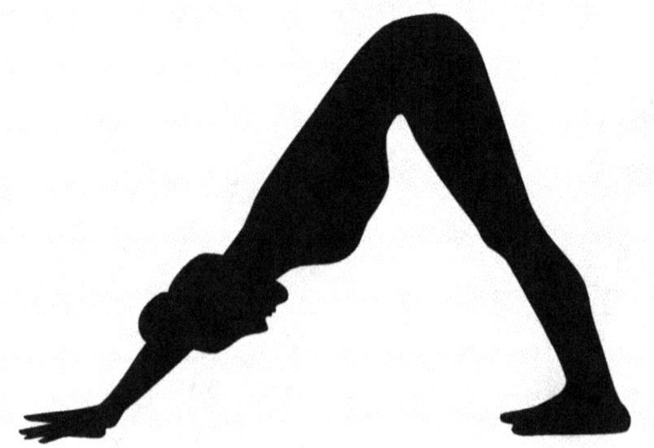

Types of Self Care

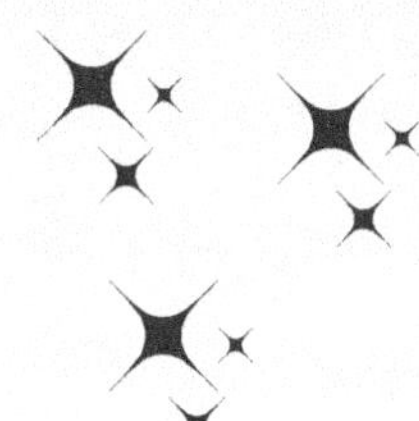

Physical Self Care

Emotional Self Care

Spiritual Self Care

Personal Self Care

Intellectual Self Care

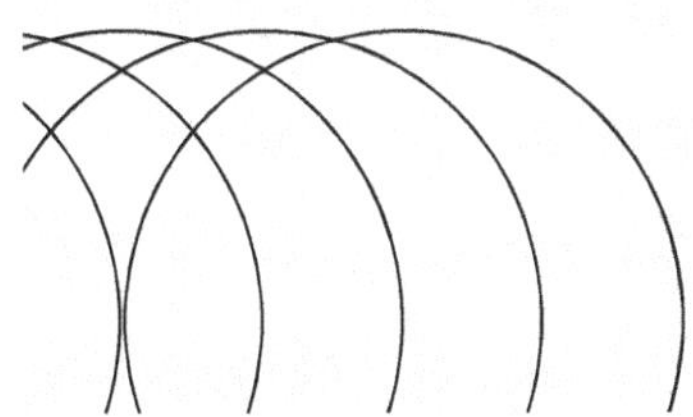

NOTES

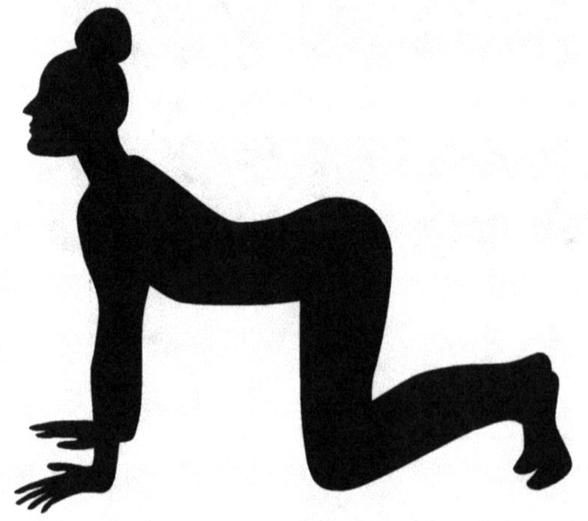

NOTES

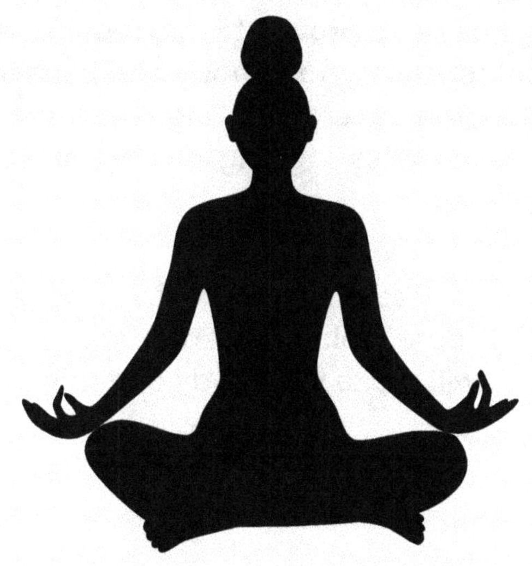

Ways to Improve Self Care

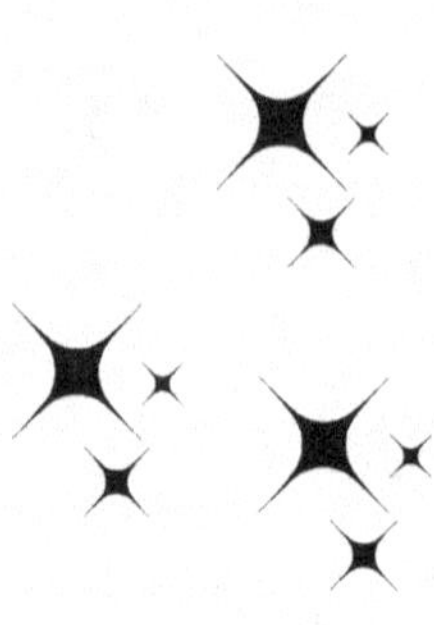

INCREASE SELF ESTEEM

Self esteem is the most important part of self care, especially in avoiding psychiatric or psychological illness. This is because a low level of self-esteem can put oneself in a state of constant anxiety and negative thinking.

MEDITATION

Meditating will help you to recognize emotional feelings, whether they are positive or negative emotions. Spend at least 5-10 minutes a day meditating.

EXERCISING ROUTINE

Doing sports has been proven to affect our body and mind. Sports are not always synonymous with burdensome activities. There are several relaxing sports that we can apply, such as aerobics, jogging, cycling, and the like.

BODY CARE

If your body feels tired from the work you have done all day, do this self care. Doing massage, spa, or just doing aromatherapy will make your body and mind relaxed and fresh.

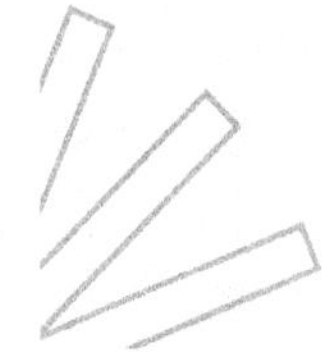

NOTES

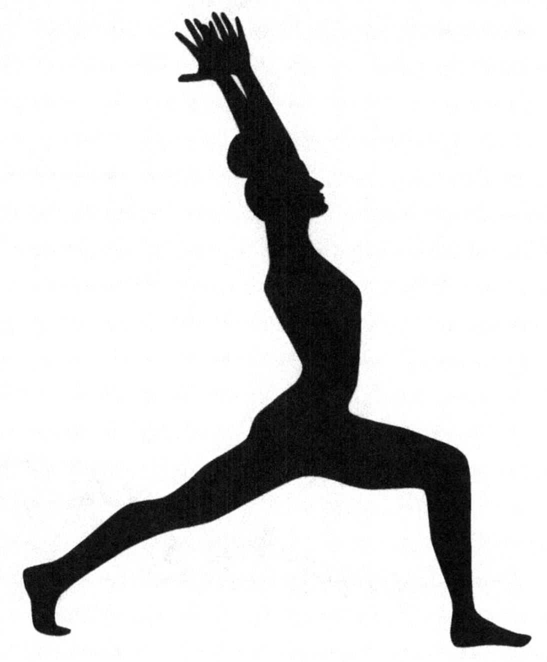

NOTES

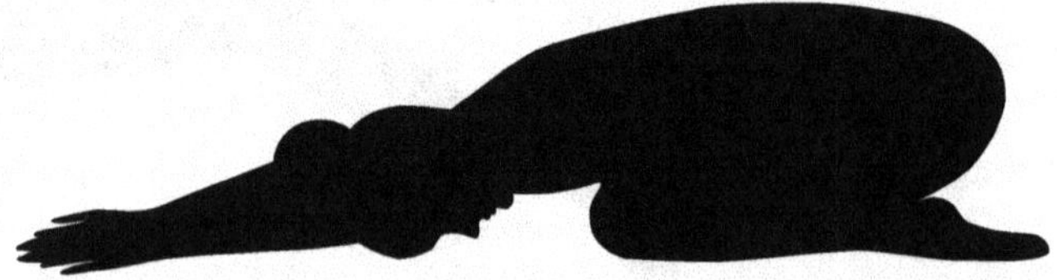

Self care Ideas for life Balance

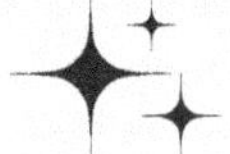

1. Take a random day off. Have a day off without any planning or purpose. Just to be off from work.
2. Plan for a weekend holiday. Go for a short trip. Escape from the routine.
3. Get to work early. Avoid the rush hour. This also means you might be able to leave work early.
4. Leave work early. Enjoy some free time when the sun is still there.
5. Eat lunch away from your office. Take a little break. Breathe some fresh air.
6. Have a small chat. Talk about something other than work. This makes your time at work less dull.
7. Turn off work-related email notification. Make off-hour really off-hour.
8. Wear your favorite outfit to work. Boost your happiness by a smart and refreshing appearance.
9. Have some healthy snacks. Supply energy to your body.
10. Listen to soft music. Relieve your stress with a soft background music.

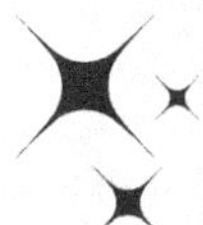

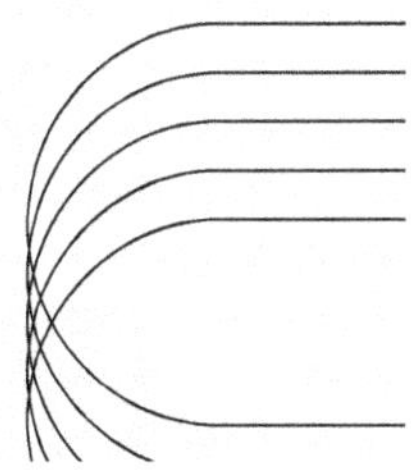

NOTES

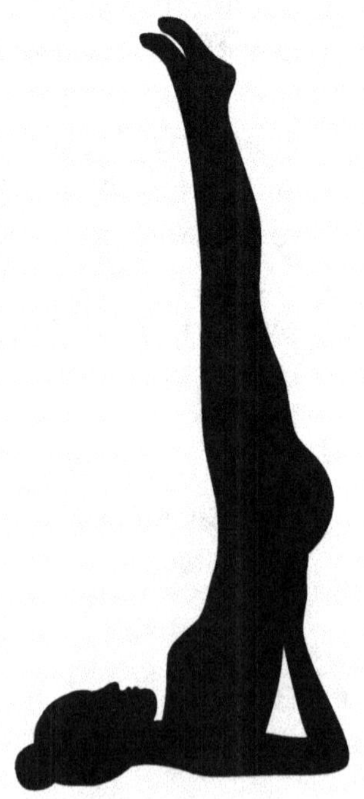

NOTES

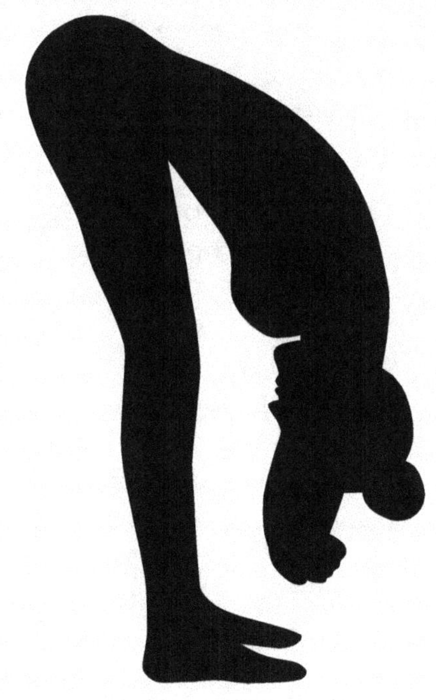

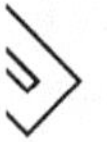
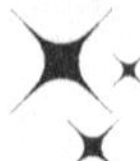

Self Care in Difficult Times

SET BOUNDARIES

On a daily basis, Ricketts recommended to, "Acknowledge your privilege, set boundaries, and learn to say no." Setting boundaries is essential to a healthy life, but it's a skill that many of us never learn.

Meditate

There's a reason that meditation is one of the most talked-about practices in the wellness world—this is powerful. Meditation is effective for self-care because it takes our focus off of the world around us, and puts it back on ourselves.

Rest (no, not just sleeping)

On a daily basis, Ricketts recommended to, "Acknowledge your privilege, set boundaries, and learn to say no." Setting boundaries is essential to a healthy life, but it's a skill that many of us never learn.

Check in with yourself frequently

There's a reason that meditation is one of the most talked-about practices in the wellness world—this sh*t is powerful. Meditation is effective for self-care because it takes our focus off of the world around us, and puts it back on ourselves.

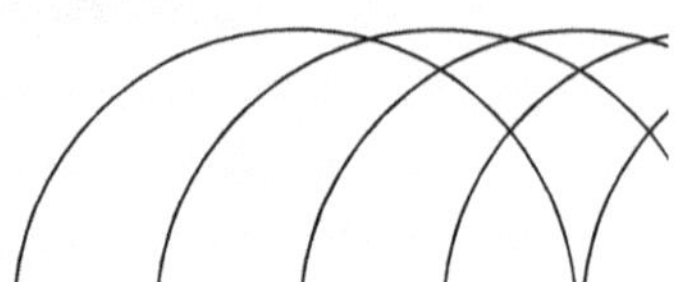

NOTES

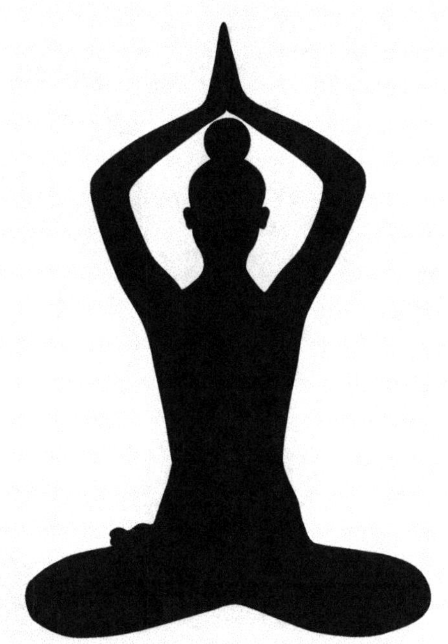

NOTES

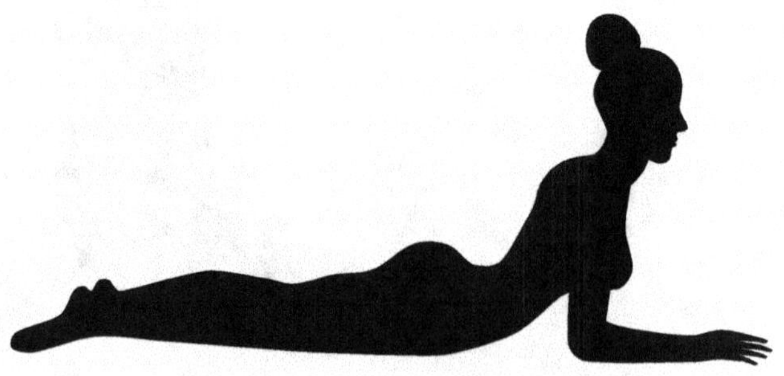

NOTES

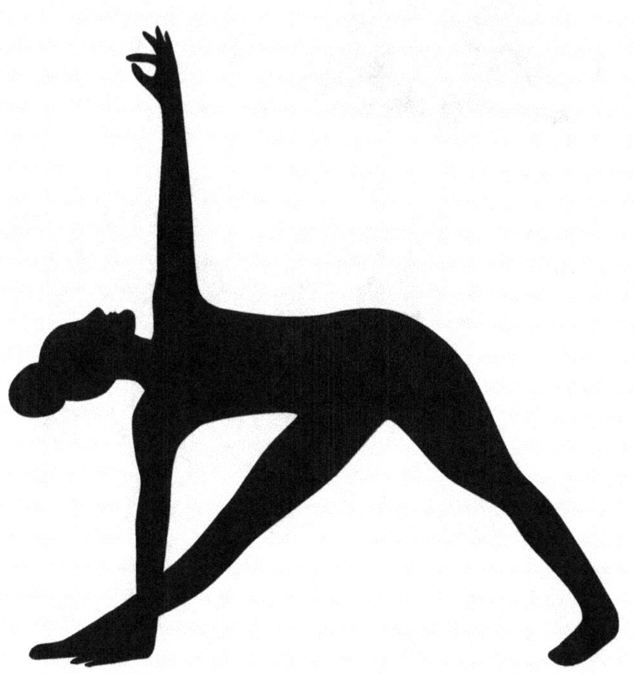

Introducing Sharon McLarin:
Advocating Self-Care for Women
Meet Sharon McLarin, a passionate
educator on the importance of self-
care for women. As mothers and
wives, it's easy to overlook our own
self-care needs amid the daily
challenges of life, which can be quite
overwhelming.

Advocating Against Domestic
Violence.

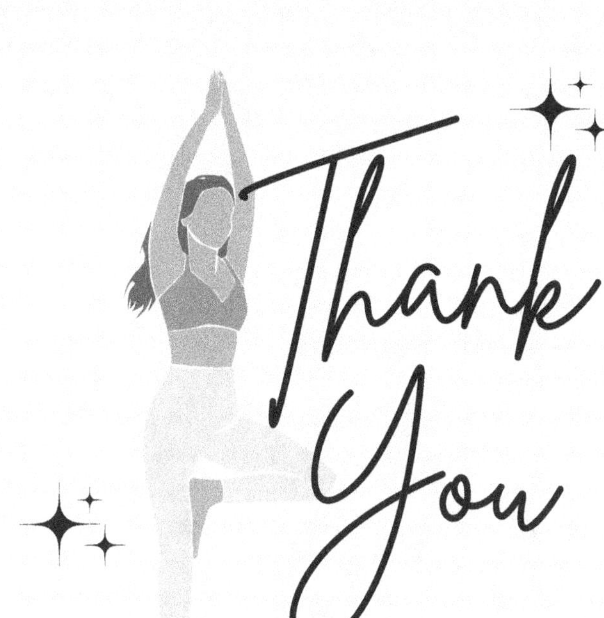

GREETINGS FROM

SHARON MCLAURIN

mclaurinsharon1@gmail.com

SHARONMCLAURIN.COM

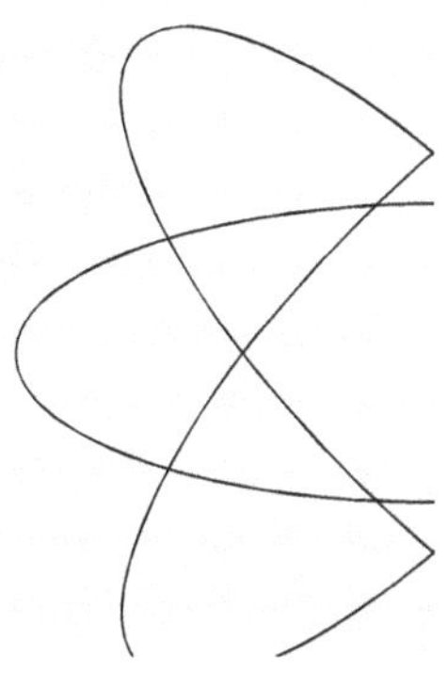